I0705236

Fertility Diet Cookbook

Boost Your Fertility Naturally with Delicious and Nutritious Recipes

Samantha Jameson

All rights reserved. No part of this publication may be reproduced, distributed, or transmitted in any form or by any means, including photocopying, recording, or other electronic or mechanical methods, without the prior written permission of the publisher, except in the case of brief quotations embodied in critical reviews and certain other noncommercial uses permitted by copyright law.

Copyright © Samantha Jameson 2023.

Table of Contents

Introduction

Chapter 1

Chapter 2 : Breakfast Recipes

3. Tropical Paradise Fertility Smoothie

4. Quinoa Breakfast Bowl

5. Oatmeal Breakfast Bowl

6. Brown Rice Breakfast Bowl

7. Spinach and Feta Omelette

8. Avocado Egg Toast

9. Berry Oatmeal Muffins

10.   Sweet Potato Muffins

Chapter 3 : Lunch Recipes

1. Quinoa and roasted vegetable salad with avocado dressing

2. Spinach, beet and goat cheese salad with citrus vinaigrette

3. Grilled chicken, avocado and black bean salad with cilantro lime dressing

4. Quinoa and Vegetable Bowl

5. Chickpea and Avocado Bowl

6. Salmon and Brown Rice Bowl

7. Grilled chicken and avocado sandwich on whole grain bread

8. Tuna salad sandwich made with Greek yogurt and topped with spinach on sprouted grain bread

9. Tomato and red pepper soup with quinoa and black beans

10. Lentil soup with spinach and carrot

Chapter 4: Dinner Recipes

1. One-Pot Quinoa and Vegetable Stir Fry

2. One-Pot Lentil and Sweet Potato Curry

3. One-Pot Salmon and Asparagus Bake

4. Quinoa and Black Bean Bowl

5. Lentil Soup

6. Veggie Stir-Fry

7. Grilled Salmon with Avocado Salsa

8. Shrimp and Spinach Pasta

9. Grilled steak with roasted sweet potatoes and asparagus

10. Pan-seared salmon with quinoa and roasted vegetables

Chapter 5 : Snack Recipes

1. Almond and date energy balls with maca powder

2. Dark chocolate and chia seed energy balls with goji berries

3. Peanut butter and honey energy balls with flaxseed meal

4. Avocado Dip

5. Beetroot Hummus

6. Spinach and Artichoke Dip

Chapter 6: Dessert Recipes

Chapter 7

1. Meal Plans for Fertility
2. Tips for meal planning and preparation

Conclusion

1. Final thoughts on the fertility diet

Introduction

Welcome to the Fertility Diet Cookbook - the ultimate guide to boosting your fertility naturally through delicious and nutritious recipes! This cookbook is a must-have for anyone who is trying to conceive and wants to optimize their chances of getting pregnant.

Filled with advice and easy-to-follow recipes, this cookbook is designed to help you make healthy food choices that will support your reproductive health. Whether you're looking for breakfast ideas, main dishes, snacks, or desserts, this cookbook has something for everyone.

Each recipe is packed with fertility-boosting ingredients that have been carefully selected to help improve your chances of conceiving. From superfoods like leafy greens, berries, and nuts to hormone-balancing ingredients like omega-3 fatty acids and antioxidants, every recipe is designed to support your fertility journey.

So whether you're just starting out on your fertility journey or looking for new and delicious ways to support your reproductive health, the Fertility Diet Cookbook is the perfect resource for you. Get ready to indulge in tasty and nutritious meals that will help you reach your ultimate goal of starting or expanding your family!

What is a fertility diet?

A fertility diet is a nutritional approach that is aimed at optimizing the reproductive health and improving the chances of conception for both men and women. It emphasizes the intake of nutrient-dense foods that are rich in vitamins, minerals, and antioxidants that are essential for fertility and pregnancy. The fertility diet is not a specific diet plan but rather a set of dietary guidelines that are based on scientific evidence and research.

The fertility diet encourages a healthy and balanced diet that includes a variety of foods from all the major food groups, such as fruits, vegetables, whole grains, lean proteins, and healthy fats. It also recommends the intake of certain foods that are known to boost fertility, such as:

Plant-based proteins: Legumes, nuts, seeds, and tofu are rich sources of plant-based proteins that are beneficial for fertility.

Fruits and vegetables: These are packed with essential vitamins and minerals, such as vitamin C, beta-carotene, and folate, which are essential for fertility.

Whole grains: Whole grains such as oats, quinoa, and brown rice are high in fiber, which is essential for maintaining hormonal balance and insulin levels.

Healthy fats: These include omega-3 fatty acids, found in oily fish like salmon and mackerel, as well as in nuts and seeds.

Antioxidant-rich foods: These are found in colorful fruits and vegetables, such as berries, leafy greens, and peppers, and help to protect against cellular damage caused by free radicals.

In addition to a healthy diet, the fertility diet also recommends avoiding certain foods and substances that can negatively impact fertility, such as:

Processed and refined foods: These are high in sugar and unhealthy fats, which can contribute to insulin resistance and hormonal imbalances.

Caffeine: High levels of caffeine consumption can interfere with fertility by disrupting the ovulation cycle.

Alcohol: Excessive alcohol consumption can lower the chances of conception and increase the risk of miscarriage.

Trans fats: These are commonly found in fast foods and fried foods and have been linked to infertility.

Smoking: Smoking can harm both male and female fertility by reducing sperm count and damaging the female reproductive system.

Overall, the fertility diet is a way of eating that emphasizes the importance of a healthy, nutrient-dense diet for optimizing reproductive health and increasing the chances of conception. It is an evidence-based approach that can help couples who are trying to conceive, and it is important to note that while it is not a guarantee of success, it can significantly improve the odds of achieving a healthy pregnancy.

The role of nutrition in fertility

Nutrition plays a critical role in fertility. Good nutrition is important for both men and women who are trying to conceive. The quality and quantity of nutrients in the body can affect the reproductive health of individuals. Here are some ways in which nutrition can impact fertility:

Nutrients for egg and sperm quality: Good nutrition is essential for the production of healthy eggs and sperm. The body requires a variety of vitamins, minerals, and other nutrients to support the development of healthy eggs and sperm. For instance, studies have shown that zinc, folic acid, and omega-3 fatty acids can improve sperm quality.

Hormone balance: Proper nutrition is also essential for maintaining hormone balance. Hormonal imbalances can affect ovulation and menstrual cycles in women and decrease sperm production in men. For example, vitamin D plays a crucial role in regulating the production of reproductive hormones in both men and women.

Body weight and fertility: Maintaining a healthy weight is important for fertility. Both being underweight or overweight can disrupt hormone balance and interfere with ovulation and sperm production. A balanced diet rich in nutrients can help individuals achieve and maintain a healthy weight.

Reducing oxidative stress: Oxidative stress occurs when there is an imbalance between the production of free radicals and the body's ability to fight them off. This can lead to damage to the DNA in the reproductive cells, which can result in infertility or miscarriage. Antioxidants like vitamins C and E can help neutralize free radicals and reduce oxidative stress.

Improving the uterine environment: A healthy uterine environment is essential for implantation and successful pregnancy. Proper nutrition can help create a healthy uterine environment by improving blood flow to the uterus, supporting the growth of the uterine lining, and reducing inflammation.

In conclusion, good nutrition is crucial for fertility. Eating a well-balanced diet rich in nutrients can help improve egg and sperm quality, regulate hormone balance, maintain a healthy weight, reduce oxidative stress, and improve the uterine environment. Individuals who are trying to conceive should pay attention to their diet and make healthy choices to optimize their chances of successful pregnancy.

Benefits of a fertility diet

A fertility diet is a type of eating plan that promotes reproductive health and improves the chances of conception. This diet focuses on consuming nutrient-rich foods, healthy fats, and adequate protein, while avoiding processed foods and trans fats.

Here are some of the benefits of a fertility diet:

Improved fertility: A healthy and balanced diet can improve fertility by regulating ovulation and promoting healthy sperm production. A fertility diet can provide the necessary nutrients and antioxidants needed to improve egg and sperm quality.

Reduced risk of ovulatory disorders: Certain foods can cause hormonal imbalances, leading to ovulatory disorders like PCOS. A fertility diet can help reduce the risk of these disorders and improve the chances of conception.

Reduced inflammation: Inflammation can have a negative impact on fertility. A fertility diet includes foods that are anti-inflammatory, such as fruits and vegetables, nuts, and omega-3 fatty acids. This can help reduce inflammation and improve reproductive health.

Reduced risk of miscarriage: Nutrient deficiencies can increase the risk of miscarriage. A fertility diet can provide the necessary vitamins and minerals needed to maintain a healthy pregnancy and reduce the risk of miscarriage.

Improved overall health: A fertility diet can improve overall health by reducing the risk of chronic diseases such as diabetes, high blood pressure, and obesity. These conditions can also have a negative impact on fertility.

In conclusion, a fertility diet can improve reproductive health, reduce the risk of ovulatory disorders and inflammation, and improve overall health. It is important to consult with a healthcare provider before making any significant dietary changes.

Chapter 1

1. Whole grains: brown rice, quinoa, bulgur, farro, oats, barley, etc.
2. Legumes: lentils, chickpeas, black beans, kidney beans, navy beans, etc.
3. Nuts: almonds, walnuts, cashews, pecans, pistachios, etc.
4. Seeds: pumpkin seeds, sunflower seeds, flaxseeds, chia seeds, sesame seeds, etc.
5. Nut butters: almond butter, peanut butter, cashew butter, etc.

6. Olive oil: extra-virgin olive oil for cooking and dressings.

7. Coconut oil: for cooking and baking.

8. Apple cider vinegar: for dressings and marinades.

9. Balsamic vinegar: for dressings and marinades.

10. Tamari or soy sauce: for flavoring stir-fries and marinades.

11. Canned tomatoes: for soups, stews, and sauces.

12. Tomato paste: for adding depth of flavor to sauces.

13. Canned beans: for quick and easy meals.

14. Canned tuna or salmon: for a quick and easy source of protein.

15. Dried fruits: raisins, apricots, dates, figs, etc. for a natural sweetener.

16.Raw honey: for natural sweetness.

17.Maple syrup: for natural sweetness.

18.   Unsweetened coconut flakes: for adding texture and flavor to baked goods or smoothies.

19.Rolled oats: for making oatmeal, granola, and baked goods.

20.   Cinnamon: for flavoring baked goods and oatmeal.

21.Ginger: for flavoring soups, stews, and stir-fries.

22.   Turmeric: for its anti-inflammatory properties.

23.   Nutritional yeast: for a cheesy flavor and a source of vitamin B12.

24.   Whole-grain pasta: for a quick and easy meal.

25.   Brown rice pasta: for a gluten-free option.

26. Quinoa pasta: for a high-protein, gluten-free option.

27. Marinara sauce: for topping pasta and pizza.

28. Pesto: for topping pasta and pizza.

29. Salsa: for topping tacos and burrito bowls.

30. Hot sauce: for adding flavor and heat to meals.

31. Chicken or vegetable broth: for making soups and stews.

32. Quinoa: for a high-protein grain.

33. Rice noodles: for making stir-fries and soups.

34. Coconut milk: for making curries and smoothies.

35. Frozen fruits: for smoothies and baking.

36. Frozen vegetables: for adding to soups and stir-fries.

37. Dark chocolate: for a healthy source of antioxidants.

38. Popcorn kernels: for a healthy snack.

39. Tea: green tea, chamomile tea, peppermint tea, etc.

40. Spices: cumin, coriander, paprika, smoked paprika, garlic powder, onion powder, etc.

41. Apple sauce: for a natural sweetener and for baking.

42. Vinegar: white vinegar, red wine vinegar, rice vinegar, etc.

43. Mustard: for dressings and marinades.

44. Ketchup: for dipping and flavoring.

45.   Almond milk: for a non-dairy milk option.

46.   Herbal supplements: red raspberry leaf, maca root, etc.

47.   Protein powder: for smoothies and baked goods.

48.   Greek yogurt: for a high-protein dairy option.

49.   Eggs: for a source of protein.

50.   Fresh fruits and vegetables: for snacking, baking, and cooking.

Kitchen equipment to help you cook nutritious meals

Steamer: A steamer is a must-have in any kitchen if you are trying to eat healthily.

Steaming your vegetables and other foods is one of the healthiest ways to cook them, as it preserves the nutrients that are often lost through other cooking methods. You can steam anything from broccoli, carrots, green beans, to fish and poultry.

Slow Cooker: A slow cooker can help you make nutritious and delicious meals with minimal effort. You can use it to cook stews, soups, and other meals that require long cooking times, which are great for fertility diets. You can use it to make bone broth or cook whole grains such as brown rice, quinoa, and oats.

Food Processor: A food processor is essential for making homemade sauces, dips, and spreads. With a food processor, you can make your own pesto, hummus, nut butter, and salad dressings. You can also chop vegetables quickly, which is great when you are in a hurry.

Blender: A blender is perfect for making smoothies, which are a great way to get all your nutrients in one meal. You can add fruits, vegetables, and protein powder to your smoothies, which are all great for fertility. You can also use a blender to make healthy soups and purees.

Non-stick frying pan: A non-stick frying pan is a great kitchen equipment to help you cook nutritious meals. You can cook eggs, poultry, and fish with very little oil or butter, which is great for fertility diets. You can also cook vegetables and grains in a non-stick pan without the need for extra fat.

Air fryer: An air fryer is a great way to cook your food without using too much oil. You can use an air fryer to cook vegetables, chicken, fish, and other foods that are great for fertility. Air fryers are also very convenient and easy to use.

Spiralizer: A spiralizer is perfect for making noodles from vegetables, such as zucchini, carrots, and sweet potatoes. You can use spiralized vegetables in place of regular pasta, which is great for fertility diets. You can also use a spiralizer to make vegetable ribbons for salads and other dishes.

Oven: An oven is essential for baking and roasting. You can use it to roast vegetables, chicken, and fish, which are great for fertility. You can also bake healthy treats, such as muffins, cookies, and cakes, using wholesome ingredients such as whole grain flours and natural sweeteners.

Chapter 2

1. Berry Blast Fertility Smoothie

Ingredients:

- 1 cup frozen mixed berries
- 1 banana
- 1/2 cup Greek yogurt
- 1/2 cup almond milk
- 1 tbsp honey
- 1 tsp maca powder

Nutritional value per serving (makes 2 servings):

Calories: 194

Carbohydrates: 38g

Protein: 7g

Fat: 2g

Fiber: 6g

Vitamin C: 78% daily value

Calcium: 16% daily value

Iron: 7% daily value

Instructions:

- Add all ingredients to a blender and blend until smooth.
- Pour into two glasses and serve immediately.

Note: This smoothie is a great source of antioxidants, vitamins, and minerals that can support fertility and reproductive health. It's also a tasty and refreshing way to start your day or to enjoy as a snack.

2. Green Goddess Fertility Smoothie

Ingredients:

- 1 cup unsweetened almond milk
- 1 ripe banana
- 1 cup frozen pineapple chunks
- 1 cup fresh spinach leaves
- 1 tablespoon ground flaxseed
- 1 teaspoon honey (optional)

Directions:

In a blender, add the almond milk, banana, frozen pineapple chunks, spinach leaves, ground flaxseed, and honey (if using).

Blend on high speed for 30-60 seconds or until the mixture is smooth and creamy.

Pour the smoothie into a glass and enjoy!

Nutritional Value:

This Green Goddess Fertility Smoothie is packed with fertility-boosting nutrients. It is an excellent source of vitamin C, which is important for both male and female fertility. The spinach leaves provide a good amount of iron, which is essential for healthy ovulation and sperm production. The ground flaxseed is a rich source of omega-3 fatty acids, which are crucial for hormonal balance and reproductive health. Plus, the banana and pineapple chunks add natural sweetness and a dose of energy-boosting carbohydrates.

Serving Size:

This recipe makes one serving. It is best to consume the smoothie immediately after blending to ensure maximum nutrient retention.

Note: While this smoothie is a healthy addition to a balanced diet, it is not a magic solution for fertility issues. Consult with your healthcare provider if you have concerns about your fertility or are trying to conceive.

3. Tropical Paradise Fertility Smoothie

Ingredients:

1 cup fresh mango chunks

1/2 cup fresh pineapple chunks

1 banana

1 cup coconut milk

1 tablespoon chia seeds

1 tablespoon honey

Nutritional value per serving:

Calories: 389

Fat: 19g

Carbohydrates: 58g

Fiber: 9g

Protein: 4g

Vitamin C: 147% of the Daily Value (DV)

Vitamin A: 41% of the DV

Calcium: 8% of the DV

Iron: 18% of the DV

Serving size: This recipe makes 2 servings.

Note: This fertility smoothie is not only delicious, but also packed with nutrients that are beneficial for reproductive health. Mango, pineapple, and banana are all rich in vitamins and minerals that support ovulation and sperm production. Coconut milk provides healthy fats that are essential for hormone balance, and chia seeds offer fiber and omega-3s that improve fertility. The addition of honey adds a touch of natural sweetness while also providing antioxidants. Enjoy this tropical paradise fertility smoothie as a healthy and tasty way to boost your fertility!

4. Quinoa Breakfast Bowl

Ingredients:

- 1 cup cooked quinoa
- 1/2 avocado, sliced
- 1/2 cup cherry tomatoes, halved
- 1/4 cup crumbled feta cheese
- 1/4 cup chopped fresh parsley
- 2 tablespoons lemon juice
- Salt and pepper to taste

Directions:

- In a bowl, mix together the cooked quinoa, sliced avocado, cherry tomatoes, crumbled feta cheese, and chopped fresh parsley.
- Drizzle with lemon juice and sprinkle with salt and pepper to taste.
- Serve immediately.

Nutritional value (per serving):

Calories: 358

Protein: 12g

Fat: 18g

Carbohydrates: 40g

Fiber: 9g

Sugar: 2g

Sodium: 277mg

Serving size: This recipe makes one serving.

Note: This quinoa breakfast bowl is a great way to start your day with a healthy and filling meal. Quinoa is a great source of protein and fiber, while the avocado adds healthy fats and the cherry tomatoes provide some vitamin C. This recipe can be easily customized with additional toppings or seasonings to suit your taste preferences.

5. Oatmeal Breakfast Bowl

Ingredients:

- 1/2 cup rolled oats
- 1 cup unsweetened almond milk
- 1 tablespoon chia seeds
- 1/2 teaspoon cinnamon
- 1/2 banana, sliced

- 1 tablespoon honey
- 1/4 cup chopped nuts (such as almonds, pecans, or walnuts)
- Fresh fruit (such as berries or sliced apples) for topping

Instructions:

- In a small pot, bring the almond milk to a simmer.
- Add in the rolled oats, chia seeds, and cinnamon. Stir well.
- Reduce heat to medium-low and let the mixture simmer for 5-7 minutes until the oats have absorbed most of the liquid.
- Remove from heat and transfer to a bowl.
- Top with sliced banana, chopped nuts, honey, and fresh fruit.

Nutritional Value:

Serving size: 1 bowl

Calories: 450

Fat: 20g

Carbohydrates: 59g

Fiber: 12g

Protein: 12g

Note:

This oatmeal breakfast bowl is high in fiber and protein, making it a satisfying and healthy breakfast option. It's also easily customizable - feel free to swap in different fruits or nuts based on your preferences.

6. Brown Rice Breakfast Bowl

Ingredients:

- 1 cup cooked brown rice

- 2 eggs

- 1 avocado, sliced

- 1/4 cup diced tomatoes

- 1/4 cup black beans

- 1/4 cup diced red onions

- 1/4 cup shredded cheddar cheese

- Salt and pepper to taste

Directions:

- In a skillet, fry 2 eggs to your desired doneness and set aside.

- In a bowl, combine cooked brown rice, black beans, diced red onions, diced tomatoes, and avocado.

- Top with the fried eggs and sprinkle with shredded cheddar cheese.

- Add salt and pepper to taste.

Nutritional Value (per serving):

Calories: 517

Protein: 22g

Fat: 30g

Carbohydrates: 42g

Fiber: 12g

Sugar: 3g

Sodium: 320mg

Serving size: This recipe makes 2 servings.

Note: This Brown Rice Breakfast Bowl is a great way to start your day off with a healthy and filling meal. It's packed with protein, fiber, healthy fats, and complex carbohydrates, making it a balanced meal that will keep you satisfied until your next meal. You can also customize this recipe by adding your favorite toppings or swapping out ingredients to suit your taste. Enjoy!

7. Spinach and Feta Omelette

Ingredients:

- 2 eggs
- 1/4 cup of fresh spinach, roughly chopped
- 1/4 cup of crumbled feta cheese
- 1 tablespoon of olive oil
- Salt and pepper to taste

Instructions:

In a small bowl, whisk the eggs until well combined. Add salt and pepper to taste.

In a non-stick skillet, heat the olive oil over medium heat. Add the chopped spinach and cook for 1-2 minutes, stirring occasionally.

Pour the eggs over the spinach and let cook for 1-2 minutes, or until the eggs begin to set.

Sprinkle the crumbled feta cheese over one half of the omelette.

Use a spatula to carefully fold the other half of the omelette over the cheese. Let cook for an additional 1-2 minutes, or until the cheese is melted and the eggs are fully cooked.

Slide the omelette onto a plate and serve hot.

Nutritional Information (per serving):

Calories: 240

Total fat: 19g

Saturated fat: 7g

Cholesterol: 370mg

Sodium: 470mg

Total carbohydrates: 2g

Dietary fiber: 0g

Sugars: 1g

Protein: 16g

Serving size: 1 omelette

Note: This Spinach and Feta Omelette is a great option for a protein-packed breakfast or lunch. It's high in protein and healthy fats, and low in carbohydrates, making it a filling and satisfying meal that won't leave you feeling sluggish. Feel free to customize the recipe with additional vegetables or herbs to suit your tastes.

8. Avocado Egg Toast

Ingredients:

- 1 slice whole-grain bread
- 1/2 medium avocado, mashed
- 1 large egg
- Salt and pepper to taste
- Optional toppings: sliced tomatoes, microgreens, hot sauce

Directions:

- Toast the bread to your desired level of crispiness.
- While the bread is toasting, cook the egg to your liking (poached, fried, or scrambled).
- Spread the mashed avocado onto the toasted bread.

- Place the cooked egg on top of the avocado, and sprinkle with salt and pepper to taste.
- Add any optional toppings you desire, and serve.

Nutritional Information (per serving):

Calories: 291

Total Fat: 20g

Saturated Fat: 4g

Cholesterol: 186mg

Sodium: 235mg

Total Carbohydrates: 19g

Dietary Fiber: 8g

Sugars: 2g

Protein: 12g

Note: This recipe makes one serving. Avocado Egg Toast is a great breakfast or brunch option that provides a balance of protein, healthy fats, and fiber to keep you feeling full and satisfied. It is also a good source of vitamins and minerals, including vitamin C, vitamin E, vitamin K, folate, and potassium. Enjoy!

9. Berry Oatmeal Muffins

Ingredients:

- 1 cup rolled oats
- 1 cup all-purpose flour
- 1/2 cup brown sugar
- 1 teaspoon baking powder
- 1/2 teaspoon baking soda
- 1/2 teaspoon salt
- 1 cup milk

- 1/4 cup vegetable oil
- 1 egg
- 1 cup fresh or frozen berries (such as blueberries or raspberries)

Instructions:

- Preheat the oven to 375°F (190°C). Line a muffin tin with paper liners or grease the cups.
- In a large mixing bowl, combine the oats, flour, brown sugar, baking powder, baking soda, and salt.
- In a separate bowl, whisk together the milk, vegetable oil, and egg.
- Add the wet ingredients to the dry ingredients and stir until just combined.
- Gently fold in the berries.

- Spoon the batter into the prepared muffin cups, filling them about 3/4 full.
- Bake for 20-25 minutes, or until a toothpick inserted into the center of a muffin comes out clean.
- Let the muffins cool in the tin for 5 minutes before transferring them to a wire rack to cool completely.

Nutritional value per serving (1 muffin):

Calories: 190

Fat: 7g

Carbohydrates: 28g

Fiber: 2g

Protein: 4g

Note: This recipe makes 12 muffins. These berry oatmeal muffins are a great breakfast or snack option, and are packed with fiber and antioxidants from the oats and berries. They can be stored in an airtight container at room temperature for up to 3 days, or in the freezer for up to 3 months. Enjoy!

10. Sweet Potato Muffins

Ingredients:

- 1 cup mashed sweet potato
- 1/2 cup unsweetened applesauce
- 1/2 cup maple syrup
- 2 eggs
- 1 teaspoon vanilla extract
- 1 cup whole wheat flour
- 1 teaspoon baking powder
- 1/2 teaspoon baking soda

- 1/2 teaspoon salt
- 1/2 teaspoon ground cinnamon
- 1/4 teaspoon ground nutmeg
- 1/4 teaspoon ground ginger
- 1/4 cup chopped pecans (optional)

Instructions:

- Preheat the oven to 375°F and line a muffin tin with paper liners.
- In a large bowl, whisk together the sweet potato, applesauce, maple syrup, eggs, and vanilla extract until smooth.
- In a separate bowl, whisk together the flour, baking powder, baking soda, salt, cinnamon, nutmeg, and ginger.
- Add the dry ingredients to the wet ingredients and stir until just

combined. Fold in the chopped pecans, if using.

- Spoon the batter into the prepared muffin tin, filling each cup about 3/4 full.
- Bake for 20-25 minutes, or until a toothpick inserted into the center of a muffin comes out clean.
- Let the muffins cool in the tin for a few minutes, then transfer them to a wire rack to cool completely.

Nutritional Value:

Serving Size: 1 muffin

Calories: 153

Fat: 3.9g

Carbohydrates: 27.8g

Fiber: 2.6g

Protein: 3.7g

Sugar: 13.7g

Sodium: 217mg

Note: These sweet potato muffins are a healthy and delicious snack or breakfast option. They're high in fiber and protein, and contain no refined sugar. Enjoy them as a part of a balanced diet

Chapter 3

1. Quinoa and roasted vegetable salad with avocado dressing

Ingredients:

- 1 cup quinoa
- 2 cups water
- 1 small sweet potato, peeled and diced
- 1 small zucchini, diced
- 1 red bell pepper, diced

- 1 yellow onion, diced
- 2 tablespoons olive oil
- Salt and pepper to taste
- 1 avocado, peeled and pitted
- 1 garlic clove
- 2 tablespoons lime juice
- 2 tablespoons water
- 2 tablespoons olive oil
- Salt and pepper to taste
- Fresh cilantro for garnish

Directions:

- Preheat the oven to 400°F (200°C).
- Rinse the quinoa in a fine mesh strainer and place it in a medium-sized saucepan with the water. Bring to a boil over medium-high heat, reduce the heat to

low and simmer for 15-20 minutes, or until the water has been absorbed and the quinoa is tender.

- In the meantime, place the sweet potato, zucchini, bell pepper, and onion on a large baking sheet. Drizzle with the olive oil and sprinkle with salt and pepper. Roast for 20-25 minutes, or until the vegetables are tender and slightly browned.

- To make the avocado dressing, place the avocado, garlic, lime juice, water, olive oil, salt, and pepper in a blender or food processor. Blend until smooth and creamy.

- In a large bowl, mix the cooked quinoa and roasted vegetables. Pour the avocado dressing over the top and toss to combine. Garnish with fresh cilantro.

- Serve warm or chilled.

Nutritional value:

Calories: 348
Total fat: 19.5g
Saturated fat: 2.6g
Cholesterol: 0mg
Sodium: 30mg
Total carbohydrates: 40.2g
Dietary fiber: 9.6g
Sugars: 5.5g
Protein: 8g

Serving size:

This recipe makes about 4 servings.

Note:

This salad is a great source of plant-based protein, healthy fats, and fiber. It's perfect for a healthy lunch or dinner and can be enjoyed warm or cold. The avocado dressing is creamy and flavorful, and it complements the roasted vegetables and quinoa perfectly. You can also add other vegetables, such as broccoli, cauliflower, or carrots, to the salad for extra nutrients and flavor.

2. Spinach, beet and goat cheese salad with citrus vinaigrette

Ingredients:

- 4 cups baby spinach leaves
- 1 large beet, roasted and diced
- 1/4 cup crumbled goat cheese
- 1/4 cup chopped walnuts
- 2 tablespoons freshly squeezed orange juice
- 2 tablespoons freshly squeezed lemon juice
- 1 tablespoon honey
- 1/4 cup olive oil
- Salt and black pepper to taste

Directions:

- Preheat the oven to 400°F. Wash and trim the beet, wrap it in foil and bake for 45-60 minutes or until tender. Once cooled, peel and dice it into small cubes.

- In a small bowl, whisk together the orange juice, lemon juice, honey, olive oil, salt and pepper until well combined.
- In a large bowl, add the spinach leaves, roasted beets, crumbled goat cheese and chopped walnuts. Drizzle the citrus vinaigrette on top and toss everything together until well coated.
- Divide the salad into 4 servings and enjoy!

Nutritional Information:

Serving Size: 1/4 of recipe

Calories: 221

Total Fat: 17g

Saturated Fat: 3g

Cholesterol: 7mg

Sodium: 174mg

Total Carbohydrates: 15g

Dietary Fiber: 3g

Sugars: 11g

Protein: 5g

Note: This salad is packed with healthy nutrients such as vitamin A, vitamin C, iron and fiber. It makes for a perfect light lunch or side dish that can be enjoyed all year round!

3. Grilled chicken, avocado and black bean salad with cilantro lime dressing

Ingredients:

- 1 pound boneless, skinless chicken breasts
- 2 tablespoons olive oil
- 1 teaspoon garlic powder
- 1/2 teaspoon cumin
- Salt and pepper, to taste
- 2 ripe avocados, diced
- 1 can black beans, drained and rinsed
- 1 red bell pepper, diced
- 1/4 red onion, diced
- 4 cups mixed greens
- 1/4 cup fresh cilantro leaves, chopped
- Juice of 1 lime
- 1/4 cup olive oil
- 1 tablespoon honey

Directions:

- Preheat a grill or grill pan to medium-high heat.
- In a small bowl, whisk together the olive oil, garlic powder, cumin, salt, and pepper. Brush the chicken with the mixture.
- Grill the chicken for 6-8 minutes per side, or until cooked through. Let cool for a few minutes, then slice.
- In a large bowl, combine the sliced chicken, diced avocado, black beans, red bell pepper, red onion, and mixed greens.
- In a small bowl, whisk together the cilantro, lime juice, olive oil, and honey. Drizzle over the salad and toss to combine.
- Serve immediately.

Nutritional Value (per serving):

Calories: 420

Fat: 26g

Carbohydrates: 26g

Fiber: 11g

Protein: 25g

Serving Size: 4

Note: This salad is not only delicious but also packed with nutrients such as protein, fiber, healthy fats, and vitamins. It is perfect for a healthy lunch or dinner option. Enjoy!

4. Quinoa and Vegetable Bowl

Ingredients:

- 1 cup quinoa
- 2 cups water

- 1 red bell pepper, sliced
- 1 zucchini, sliced
- 1 yellow onion, sliced
- 1 tbsp olive oil
- 1 tsp paprika
- 1/2 tsp garlic powder
- Salt and pepper to taste
- Fresh parsley for garnish

Instructions:

- Rinse quinoa in a fine mesh strainer and put it in a pot with 2 cups of water. Bring to a boil and then reduce heat to low. Cover and let simmer for 15-20 minutes, or until water is absorbed and quinoa is fluffy.
- In a large skillet, heat olive oil over medium heat. Add bell pepper, zucchini, and onion. Season with

paprika, garlic powder, salt, and pepper. Cook for 10-15 minutes or until vegetables are tender.

- Divide quinoa and vegetables into serving bowls. Garnish with fresh parsley.

Nutritional Value:

Serving size: 1 bowl

Calories: 327

Fat: 8g

Carbohydrates: 53g

Fiber: 8g

Protein: 11g

Note:

This quinoa and vegetable bowl is not only delicious, but also packed with essential nutrients such as fiber, protein, and vitamins. It's a perfect meal for a healthy and balanced diet.

5. Chickpea and Avocado Bowl

Ingredients:

- 1 cup cooked chickpeas
- 1 avocado, diced
- 1 cup cherry tomatoes, halved
- 1/2 red onion, diced
- 1/4 cup chopped fresh cilantro
- 1 tablespoon olive oil
- 1 tablespoon lemon juice
- Salt and pepper to taste

Directions:

- In a large mixing bowl, combine cooked chickpeas, diced avocado, halved cherry tomatoes, diced red onion, and chopped cilantro.
- Drizzle with olive oil and lemon juice, then toss until everything is well coated.
- Season with salt and pepper to taste.
- Serve immediately, or store in an airtight container in the refrigerator for up to 3 days.

Nutritional Value (per serving):

Calories: 393

Fat: 25g

Carbohydrates: 35g

Fiber: 14g

Protein: 10g

Serving Size: This recipe makes 2-3 servings.

Note: This Chickpea and Avocado Bowl is a delicious and nutritious meal that is easy to prepare and perfect for lunch or dinner. It is a good source of fiber, healthy fats, and protein. It is also vegan, gluten-free, and dairy-free. Enjoy!

6. Salmon and Brown Rice Bowl

Ingredients:

- 1 cup brown rice
- 1 tablespoon olive oil
- 1 pound salmon filets

- 1/2 teaspoon salt

- 1/4 teaspoon black pepper

- 2 cups mixed vegetables (broccoli, carrots, bell peppers, etc.)

- 1 tablespoon soy sauce

- 1 tablespoon honey

- 1 tablespoon rice vinegar

- Sesame seeds, for garnish

Instructions:

- Cook the brown rice according to package instructions.

- Heat the olive oil in a pan over medium-high heat. Season the salmon with salt and pepper and place in the pan, skin-side down. Cook for 4-5 minutes, then flip and cook for an additional 2-3 minutes until the salmon is cooked through. Remove from pan and set aside.

- In the same pan, add the mixed vegetables and cook for 3-4 minutes until tender.

- In a small bowl, whisk together the soy sauce, honey, and rice vinegar. Pour over the vegetables and stir to coat.

- To assemble the bowls, divide the cooked brown rice between four bowls. Top with the cooked salmon and vegetables. Garnish with sesame seeds.

Nutritional value per serving (1 bowl):

Calories: 425

Fat: 16g

Saturated Fat: 2.5g

Cholesterol: 75mg

Sodium: 588mg

Carbohydrates: 40g

Fiber: 4g

Sugar: 8g

Protein: 30g

Serving size: 1 bowl

Note: This salmon and brown rice bowl is a healthy and balanced meal, packed with protein, fiber, and healthy fats. It's a great option for a quick and easy weeknight dinner, and can easily be customized with your favorite veggies or sauces.

7. Grilled chicken and avocado sandwich on whole grain bread

Ingredients:

- 2 slices of whole grain bread
- 1 grilled chicken breast
- 1/2 avocado, sliced
- 2 lettuce leaves
- 2 slices of tomato
- 1 tablespoon of mayonnaise (optional)
- Salt and pepper to taste

Instructions:

Grill the chicken breast until it's fully cooked. Slice the chicken into thin pieces.

Toast the slices of whole grain bread until they're crispy.

Spread a thin layer of mayonnaise (optional) on each slice of bread.

Add the sliced chicken breast on one slice of bread.

Top the chicken with slices of avocado, lettuce leaves, and tomato.

Season with salt and pepper to taste.

Place the other slice of bread on top.

Nutritional Information:

Serving Size: 1 sandwich

Calories: 402

Total Fat: 15g

Saturated Fat: 2.9g

Cholesterol: 70mg

Sodium: 426mg

Total Carbohydrates: 35g

Dietary Fiber: 9g

Sugars: 4g

Protein: 35g

Note: This grilled chicken and avocado sandwich is a delicious and healthy option for lunch or dinner. It's packed with protein, fiber, and healthy fats. You can adjust the serving size to meet your nutritional needs. Enjoy!

8. **Tuna salad sandwich made with Greek yogurt and topped with spinach on sprouted grain bread**

Ingredients:

- 1 can of tuna, drained and flaked
- 2 tablespoons of Greek yogurt
- 1 tablespoon of chopped red onion
- 1 tablespoon of chopped celery
- 1 tablespoon of chopped dill pickle
- 1 teaspoon of lemon juice
- Salt and pepper to taste
- 2 slices of sprouted grain bread
- A handful of baby spinach

Instructions:

- In a medium bowl, mix together tuna, Greek yogurt, red onion, celery, dill pickle, lemon juice, salt, and pepper.
- Toast the sprouted grain bread slices.
- Top one slice of the bread with the tuna salad mixture.
- Add a handful of baby spinach on top of the tuna salad.
- Close the sandwich with the other slice of bread.
- Serve and enjoy!

Nutritional Value (per serving):

Calories: 260

Fat: 5g

Carbohydrates: 27g

Protein: 26g

Fiber: 6g

Sugar: 4g

Sodium: 410mg

Serving Size:

This recipe makes 1 sandwich serving.

Note:

This tuna salad sandwich is a healthy and delicious lunch option that is packed with protein and fiber. It is a great source of omega-3 fatty acids and essential nutrients that can help support a balanced diet. Sprouted grain bread is a nutrient-dense option that provides more vitamins and minerals compared to traditional bread. Enjoy this tasty sandwich as a quick and easy meal on busy days!

9. Lentil soup with spinach and carrot

Ingredients:

- 1 cup green lentils
- 1 onion, chopped
- 2 garlic cloves, minced
- 2 carrots, chopped
- 4 cups vegetable broth
- 1 tsp ground cumin
- 1 tsp ground coriander
- 2 cups fresh spinach leaves
- Salt and pepper to taste
- Olive oil

Directions:

- In a large pot, heat olive oil over medium heat. Add chopped onions and sauté until softened, about 5 minutes. Add garlic and cook for an additional minute.

- Add chopped carrots, lentils, vegetable broth, cumin, and coriander to the pot. Bring to a boil, then reduce heat and let simmer for 25-30 minutes or until the lentils are tender.
- Add fresh spinach to the pot and stir until wilted. Season with salt and pepper to taste.
- Serve hot and enjoy!

Nutritional Information (per serving):

Calories: 226

Fat: 2g

Carbohydrates: 38g

Fiber: 16g

Protein: 14g

Serving Size: This recipe yields approximately 4 servings.

Note: Lentil soup is a great source of plant-based protein and fiber. Spinach adds extra nutrients like iron, vitamin C, and vitamin K. This recipe is a delicious and healthy option for a warm and satisfying meal.

10. Tomato and red pepper soup with quinoa and black beans

Ingredients:

- 2 red peppers, deseeded and chopped
- 1 onion, chopped

- 3 cloves garlic, minced
- 1 can diced tomatoes
- 4 cups vegetable broth
- 1/2 cup quinoa
- 1 can black beans, rinsed and drained
- 1 tsp cumin
- 1 tsp paprika
- Salt and pepper, to taste
- 1 tbsp olive oil

Instructions:

- In a large pot, heat olive oil over medium-high heat. Add onion and cook until softened, about 5 minutes.
- Add garlic, cumin, paprika, and red peppers. Cook for another 5 minutes.
- Pour in diced tomatoes and vegetable broth. Bring to a boil, then reduce heat and let simmer for 20 minutes.

- Add quinoa and black beans to the pot. Cook for another 15-20 minutes, or until quinoa is fully cooked.
- Season with salt and pepper to taste.
- Serve hot and enjoy!

Nutritional Value (per serving):

Calories: 250

Fat: 6g

Carbohydrates: 42g

Fiber: 12g

Protein: 10g

Serving Size:

This recipe serves 4 people.

Note:

This soup is not only delicious but also packed with nutrients. Quinoa and black beans provide a good source of protein and fiber, while red peppers and tomatoes are rich in vitamins and antioxidants. Enjoy this soup as a complete meal or pair it with a fresh salad for a satisfying and healthy lunch or dinner.

Chapter 4

Dinner Recipes

1. One-Pot Quinoa and Vegetable Stir Fry

Ingredients:

- 1 cup uncooked quinoa
- 1 tablespoon olive oil
- 1 small onion, diced
- 2 garlic cloves, minced

- 2 cups mixed vegetables (e.g. broccoli, bell peppers, snap peas, carrots)
- 2 cups vegetable broth
- 1 tablespoon soy sauce
- Salt and pepper, to taste
- Chopped green onions and sesame seeds, for garnish

Directions:

- Rinse quinoa under cold water and drain.
- In a large pot or deep skillet, heat olive oil over medium-high heat. Add onions and garlic and sauté for 2-3 minutes, or until onions are translucent.
- Add mixed vegetables and stir fry for 5-7 minutes, or until vegetables are tender.

- Add quinoa, vegetable broth, and soy sauce. Stir well and bring to a boil.
- Reduce heat to low, cover and simmer for 15-20 minutes or until quinoa is fully cooked.
- Season with salt and pepper to taste. Garnish with chopped green onions and sesame seeds before serving.

Nutrition per serving (1 cup):

Calories: 202

Fat: 5.5g

Saturated Fat: 0.8g

Carbohydrates: 31.2g

Fiber: 4.4g

Sugar: 2.4g

Protein: 7.4g

Sodium: 420mg

Serves 4.

Note: This recipe is a great source of plant-based protein and fiber, and is also vegan and gluten-free. It can be served as a main dish or as a side dish.

2. One-Pot Lentil and Sweet Potato Curry

Ingredients:

- 1 tablespoon coconut oil
- 1 onion, diced
- 2 garlic cloves, minced
- 1 tablespoon grated ginger
- 2 teaspoons curry powder
- 1 teaspoon ground cumin

- 1/2 teaspoon ground coriander
- 1/4 teaspoon cayenne pepper (optional)
- 1 large sweet potato, peeled and diced
- 1 cup red lentils, rinsed and drained
- 1 can (14 oz) diced tomatoes
- 2 cups vegetable broth
- Salt and pepper to taste
- Fresh cilantro, for garnish

Instructions:

Heat coconut oil in a large pot over medium heat. Add onion and cook for 3-5 minutes or until softened.

Add garlic, ginger, curry powder, cumin, coriander, and cayenne pepper (if using) and cook for another 2 minutes or until fragrant.

Add sweet potato, lentils, diced tomatoes, and vegetable broth. Stir well and bring to a boil.

Reduce heat to low and let simmer for 20-25 minutes or until sweet potato and lentils are tender.

Season with salt and pepper to taste. Garnish with fresh cilantro before serving.

Nutritional Information:

Serving Size: 1/6 of recipe

Calories: 234

Total Fat: 5g

Saturated Fat: 3g

Cholesterol: 0mg

Sodium: 416mg

Total Carbohydrates: 38g

Dietary Fiber: 8g

Sugars: 7g

Protein: 10g

Note: This recipe is vegan, gluten-free, and high in fiber and protein. It makes 6 servings, so feel free to freeze any leftovers for a quick and healthy meal later on. Enjoy!

3. One-Pot Salmon and Asparagus Bake

Ingredients:

- 4 salmon fillets
- 1 lb asparagus

- 1 lemon, sliced

- 4 garlic cloves, minced

- 1 tbsp olive oil

- 1 tsp dried dill

- Salt and pepper to taste

Directions:

- Preheat oven to 375°F.

- Wash and trim asparagus, then lay them out in a single layer in a baking dish.

- Place salmon fillets on top of asparagus.

- Drizzle olive oil over the salmon and asparagus.

- Sprinkle minced garlic, dried dill, salt, and pepper over the salmon.

- Place lemon slices on top of the salmon.

- Cover the baking dish with foil and bake for 20 minutes.
- Remove the foil and bake for an additional 10-15 minutes until the salmon is fully cooked.

Nutrition Facts (per serving, serves 4):

Calories: 294

Fat: 15g

Saturated Fat: 2g

Cholesterol: 79mg

Sodium: 107mg

Carbohydrates: 7g

Fiber: 3g

Sugar: 2g

Protein: 32g

Note: This One-Pot Salmon and Asparagus Bake is a great source of protein and healthy fats, and is low in calories and carbohydrates. Enjoy it as a complete meal on its own or pair it with a side of quinoa or brown rice for a more filling meal.

4. Quinoa and Black Bean Bowl

Ingredients:

- 1 cup quinoa
- 2 cups water
- 1 can black beans, drained and rinsed
- 1 red bell pepper, diced
- 1 avocado, diced
- 1 lime, juiced
- 1/4 cup chopped fresh cilantro
- Salt and pepper to taste

Instructions:

- Rinse quinoa in a fine mesh strainer and add it to a medium saucepan with 2 cups of water.

- Bring the quinoa to a boil, then reduce heat to low and simmer, covered, for 15-20 minutes or until the water is absorbed.

- In a large bowl, mix together the cooked quinoa, black beans, red bell pepper, avocado, lime juice, and cilantro.

- Season with salt and pepper to taste.

Nutritional Value:
This recipe makes approximately 4 servings.
Here is the nutritional value per serving:

Calories: 359
Total Fat: 10.3g

Saturated Fat: 1.3g

Cholesterol: 0mg

Sodium: 293mg

Total Carbohydrates: 56.3g

Dietary Fiber: 16.3g

Sugars: 3.7g

Protein: 15.5g

Note:

This quinoa and black bean bowl is a great source of protein and fiber, making it a filling and nutritious meal. It can be served as a vegetarian main dish or as a side dish to grilled chicken or fish. Leftovers can be stored in an airtight container in the fridge for up to 4 days.

5. Lentil Soup

Ingredients:

- 1 cup dry lentils
- 1 onion, chopped
- 2 cloves garlic, minced
- 1 carrot, chopped
- 1 celery stalk, chopped
- 4 cups vegetable broth
- 1 can diced tomatoes
- 1 tsp cumin
- 1 tsp coriander
- Salt and pepper to taste

Instructions:

- Rinse lentils and set aside.
- In a large pot, sauté onion and garlic until fragrant and translucent.

- Add in carrot and celery and sauté for a few more minutes.
- Pour in vegetable broth and bring to a boil.
- Add in lentils, canned tomatoes, and spices.
- Reduce heat and simmer for 30-40 minutes or until lentils are tender.
- Season with salt and pepper to taste.

Serving size: 1 cup

Nutritional Value per serving:

Calories: 177

Fat: 1g

Saturated Fat: 0g

Cholesterol: 0mg

Sodium: 517mg

Carbohydrates: 32g

Fiber: 12g

Sugar: 6g

Protein: 12g

Note: Lentil soup is a hearty and healthy meal that is packed with fiber and protein. It is a great option for vegetarians and vegans as well as those looking to reduce their meat consumption. This recipe is also low in fat and calories, making it a great addition to any weight loss diet.

6. Veggie Stir-Fry

Ingredients:

- 1 tablespoon vegetable oil
- 1 onion, sliced
- 2 cloves garlic, minced
- 1 bell pepper, sliced

- 1 zucchini, sliced

- 1 cup broccoli florets

- 1 cup snow peas

- 1 tablespoon soy sauce

- 1 tablespoon honey

- 1 teaspoon sesame oil

- 1 teaspoon grated fresh ginger

- Salt and pepper, to taste

Instructions:

- Heat the vegetable oil in a large wok or skillet over high heat.

- Add the onion and garlic and stir-fry for 1-2 minutes until fragrant.

- Add the bell pepper, zucchini, broccoli, and snow peas and stir-fry for 3-4 minutes until crisp-tender.

- In a small bowl, whisk together the soy sauce, honey, sesame oil, and ginger.

- Pour the sauce over the vegetables and stir to combine.
- Season with salt and pepper to taste.
- Serve hot with rice or noodles.

Nutritional Value per serving (makes 4 servings):

Calories: 110

Total fat: 4.5g

Saturated fat: 0.5g

Cholesterol: 0mg

Sodium: 220mg

Total carbohydrate: 16g

Dietary fiber: 4g

Sugar: 9g

Protein: 3g

Serving size: 1 cup

Note: This veggie stir-fry recipe is not only delicious but also packed with nutrients. It is a great way to add more veggies to your diet and can be customized to include your favorite vegetables. Enjoy as a main dish or as a side dish with your favorite protein.

7. Grilled Salmon with Avocado Salsa

Ingredients:

- 4 salmon fillets
- 2 avocados, diced
- 1/4 red onion, finely chopped
- 1 jalapeno pepper, seeded and finely chopped
- 1/4 cup chopped fresh cilantro

- 2 tablespoons lime juice
- Salt and pepper to taste

Instructions:

- Preheat the grill to medium-high heat.
- Season the salmon fillets with salt and pepper and grill for 5-7 minutes on each side, or until fully cooked.
- In a bowl, combine the diced avocado, red onion, jalapeno pepper, cilantro, and lime juice. Season with salt and pepper to taste.
- Serve the grilled salmon with the avocado salsa on top.

Serving size: 1 salmon fillet with 1/4 of the avocado salsa

Nutritional value per serving:

Calories: 376

Fat: 25g

Saturated Fat: 4g

Cholesterol: 76mg

Sodium: 80mg

Carbohydrates: 10g

Fiber: 7g

Sugar: 1g

Protein: 31g

Note: This recipe is not only delicious, but also a great source of healthy fats, fiber, and protein. It's perfect for a healthy and satisfying dinner that's easy to make. Enjoy!

8. Shrimp and Spinach Pasta

Ingredients:

- 8 oz. whole wheat pasta
- 1 lb. shrimp, peeled and deveined
- 2 cloves garlic, minced
- 1/4 tsp. red pepper flakes
- 1 tbsp. olive oil
- 4 cups baby spinach
- 1/2 cup cherry tomatoes, halved
- 1/4 cup grated parmesan cheese
- Salt and pepper to taste

Instructions:

- Cook the pasta according to package directions. Drain and set aside.
- In a large skillet, heat the olive oil over medium heat. Add the minced garlic and red pepper flakes and cook for 1-2 minutes.

- Add the shrimp to the skillet and cook for 3-4 minutes, or until pink and cooked through.
- Add the baby spinach and cherry tomatoes to the skillet and cook for an additional 1-2 minutes, or until the spinach has wilted.
- Add the cooked pasta to the skillet and toss to combine all the ingredients. Season with salt and pepper to taste.
- Sprinkle the grated parmesan cheese over the top of the pasta and serve hot.

Nutritional Value (per serving):

Calories: 445

Fat: 9g

Saturated Fat: 2g

Cholesterol: 245mg

Sodium: 324mg

Carbohydrates: 50g

Fiber: 9g

Sugar: 3g

Protein: 42g

Serving size: 4

Note: This dish is a great source of protein and fiber, and the whole wheat pasta adds some extra nutrients. The spinach and tomatoes also provide a serving of vegetables, making this a well-rounded meal. If you're watching your sodium intake, you can reduce the amount of salt or use a low-sodium option. Enjoy!

9. Grilled steak with roasted sweet potatoes and asparagus

Ingredients:

- 1 pound sirloin steak
- 1 teaspoon garlic powder
- 1 teaspoon onion powder
- 1 teaspoon paprika
- 1/2 teaspoon salt
- 1/4 teaspoon black pepper
- 2 sweet potatoes, peeled and cubed
- 1 bunch asparagus, trimmed
- 1 tablespoon olive oil

Instructions:

- Preheat grill to medium-high heat.

- In a small bowl, mix together garlic powder, onion powder, paprika, salt, and black pepper.
- Rub the spice mixture onto both sides of the steak.
- Grill the steak for about 6-8 minutes per side, or until desired doneness is reached.
- Meanwhile, preheat oven to 400°F.
- Toss sweet potatoes with olive oil and spread them on a baking sheet. Roast for about 20-25 minutes, or until tender and golden brown.
- In the last 10 minutes of roasting, add asparagus to the baking sheet and toss with olive oil.
- Roast for an additional 10 minutes or until asparagus is tender and lightly browned.

- Serve the grilled steak with roasted sweet potatoes and asparagus on the side.

Nutritional value (per serving):

Calories: 425

Total fat: 19g

Saturated fat: 6g

Cholesterol: 84mg

Sodium: 555mg

Total carbohydrates: 31g

Dietary fiber: 7g

Sugars: 8g

Protein: 34g

Serving size: 4

Note: This meal is high in protein and fiber, making it a satisfying and nutritious option. The sweet potatoes are a great source of vitamins A and C, while the asparagus provides folate and antioxidants. To make this meal even more balanced, consider adding a side salad or other non-starchy vegetables. Enjoy!

10. Pan-seared salmon with quinoa and roasted vegetables

Ingredients:

- 2 salmon fillets
- 1 cup quinoa
- 2 cups mixed vegetables (broccoli, bell peppers, carrots)
- 1 tbsp olive oil
- 1 tsp garlic powder

- Salt and pepper to taste
- Lemon wedges for serving

Nutritional value per serving:

Calories: 460

Protein: 36g

Carbohydrates: 41g

Fat: 18g

Fiber: 8g

Serving size: 2

Note: Quinoa is a great source of plant-based protein and fiber. The salmon provides healthy omega-3 fatty acids and protein. The mixed vegetables offer a variety of vitamins and minerals. This dish is perfect for a healthy and satisfying meal.

Instructions:

- Cook the quinoa according to package instructions and set aside.
- Preheat the oven to 400°F.
- Cut the vegetables into bite-size pieces and toss with olive oil, garlic powder, salt, and pepper. Spread the vegetables on a baking sheet and roast for 20-25 minutes, or until tender.
- Heat a large skillet over medium-high heat. Season the salmon with salt and pepper and place the fillets in the skillet, skin-side down. Cook for 5-6 minutes, or until the skin is crispy. Flip the fillets and cook for an additional 2-3 minutes, or until the salmon is cooked through.

- Divide the quinoa and roasted vegetables between two plates. Place a salmon fillet on top of each plate and serve with lemon wedges. Enjoy!

Chapter 5

Snack Recipes

1. Almond and date energy balls with maca powder

Ingredients:

- 1 cup pitted dates
- 1 cup raw almonds
- 1 tbsp maca powder
- 1 tbsp water

Directions:

- In a food processor, blend the dates and almonds until they form a sticky mixture.
- Add in the maca powder and water, and blend until everything is well combined.
- Using your hands, roll the mixture into bite-sized balls.
- Store in an airtight container in the fridge for up to 1 week.

Nutritional value (per serving, makes 12 balls):

Calories: 106

Fat: 5g

Carbohydrates: 15g

Fiber: 2g

Protein: 3g

Maca powder is known to boost energy levels and improve stamina, making these balls the perfect snack to fuel your day.
Serving size:

This recipe makes 12 energy balls, with a recommended serving size of 2 balls.
Note:

Feel free to adjust the amount of maca powder to your liking. Start with a smaller amount and gradually increase if you prefer a stronger flavor.

You can also roll the energy balls in shredded coconut or cocoa powder for an extra boost of flavor.

2. Dark chocolate and chia seed energy balls with goji berries

Ingredients:

- 1/2 cup chia seeds
- 1/2 cup goji berries
- 1/2 cup almond flour
- 1/4 cup cocoa powder
- 1/4 cup honey
- 1/4 cup coconut oil
- 1/2 cup dark chocolate chips
- 1/2 teaspoon vanilla extract

Instructions:

- In a large mixing bowl, combine the chia seeds, goji berries, almond flour, and cocoa powder.

- In a separate microwave-safe bowl, heat the honey and coconut oil for 30 seconds or until melted.
- Add the melted honey and coconut oil to the dry ingredients and mix until well combined.
- Stir in the dark chocolate chips and vanilla extract.
- Form the mixture into small balls, about 1-2 tablespoons each.
- Place the energy balls on a baking sheet lined with parchment paper and chill in the fridge for at least 30 minutes before serving.

Nutritional Value:

Serving size: 2 energy balls
Calories: 208
Total Fat: 13g

Saturated Fat: 6g

Cholesterol: 0mg

Sodium: 5mg

Total Carbohydrates: 23g

Dietary Fiber: 7g

Sugars: 12g

Protein: 4g

Note:

These energy balls are a great snack for when you need a quick energy boost. The combination of chia seeds, goji berries, and dark chocolate provides a good source of fiber, protein, and antioxidants. The serving size of 2 energy balls provides a reasonable amount of calories and can be a great addition to a balanced diet. These energy balls can be stored in an airtight container in the fridge for up to a week. Enjoy!

3. **Peanut butter and honey energy balls with flaxseed meal**

Ingredients:

- 1 cup creamy peanut butter
- 1/2 cup honey
- 1 tsp vanilla extract
- 2 cups old-fashioned oats
- 1/2 cup ground flaxseed meal
- 1/2 cup mini chocolate chips (optional)

Instructions:

- In a large bowl, mix together the peanut butter, honey, and vanilla extract until smooth.

- Add the oats, flaxseed meal, and chocolate chips (if using) to the bowl and mix until everything is well combined.
- Using a tablespoon, scoop the mixture and roll it into balls. Place the balls onto a baking sheet or plate lined with parchment paper.
- Chill the energy balls in the refrigerator for at least 30 minutes to firm up.

Nutritional Value (per serving, based on 1 energy ball):

Calories: 120

Fat: 6.6g

Saturated Fat: 1.3g

Cholesterol: 0mg

Carbohydrates: 12.8g

Fiber: 2.3g

Sugar: 6.2g

Protein: 3.7g

Serving Size: This recipe makes about 24 energy balls, and one serving is one energy ball.

Note: These Peanut Butter and Honey Energy Balls with Flaxseed Meal are a great snack option for anyone who needs a quick burst of energy. They are packed with fiber, healthy fats, and protein, and are perfect for on-the-go snacking. The recipe can be easily customized by adding in different mix-ins like raisins, chopped nuts, or dried fruit.

4. Avocado Dip

Ingredients:

- 2 ripe avocados
- 1/4 cup diced red onion
- 1/4 cup chopped fresh cilantro
- 1 small jalapeño pepper, seeded and minced
- 2 tablespoons lime juice
- Salt and pepper, to taste

Instructions:

- Cut the avocados in half, remove the pit and scoop out the flesh into a bowl.
- Mash the avocados with a fork or a potato masher.
- Add the red onion, cilantro, jalapeño pepper and lime juice. Stir well to combine.
- Season with salt and pepper, to taste.

- Cover and chill in the fridge for at least 30 minutes before serving.

Nutritional Value:

Serving size: 1/4 cup (about 60g)

Calories: 94

Fat: 8g

Saturated Fat: 1g

Cholesterol: 0mg

Sodium: 2mg

Carbohydrates: 5g

Fiber: 4g

Sugar: 0g

Protein: 1g

Note:

Avocado dip is a great addition to any party or gathering. It's also a healthy snack option, as it's high in fiber, healthy fats, and nutrients such as vitamin C, vitamin K, and folate. Serve it with veggies, tortilla chips, or pita bread for a delicious and nutritious snack. Enjoy!

5. Beetroot Hummus

Ingredients:

- 2 medium-sized beetroots, cooked and peeled
- 1 can of chickpeas, drained and rinsed
- 2 garlic cloves, chopped
- 1/4 cup of tahini
- 1/4 cup of lemon juice
- 1/4 cup of olive oil
- 1/2 teaspoon of salt

- 1/2 teaspoon of cumin
- 1/4 teaspoon of black pepper
- Water (as needed)

Instructions:

- In a food processor, combine the cooked beetroots, chickpeas, and garlic. Pulse until coarsely chopped.
- Add the tahini, lemon juice, olive oil, salt, cumin, and black pepper. Process until smooth.
- If the mixture is too thick, add water, 1 tablespoon at a time, until desired consistency is achieved.
- Taste and adjust seasoning, if needed.
- Transfer the beetroot hummus to a serving bowl and drizzle with a little more olive oil. Serve with pita chips or vegetable sticks.

Nutritional Value (per serving):

Calories: 168

Total fat: 10g

Saturated fat: 1g

Cholesterol: 0mg

Sodium: 257mg

Total carbohydrates: 17g

Dietary fiber: 4g

Sugars: 3g

Protein: 4g

Serving Size: This recipe makes about 2 cups of hummus, which can serve 6-8 people as a snack or appetizer.

Note: Beetroot hummus is a healthier alternative to traditional hummus as it is lower in calories and higher in nutrients. It is also a great source of fiber and plant-based protein. The addition of beetroot not only gives the hummus a beautiful color but also adds a unique flavor and texture. Enjoy this delicious and nutritious dip with your favorite crunchy snacks or veggies.

6. Spinach and Artichoke Dip

Ingredients:

- 10 oz. package of frozen spinach, thawed and drained
- 1 can of artichoke hearts, drained and chopped
- 8 oz. cream cheese, softened
- 1/2 cup sour cream
- 1/2 cup mayonnaise

- 1/2 cup grated Parmesan cheese
- 1/2 tsp garlic powder
- Salt and pepper to taste

Directions:

- Preheat the oven to 350°F.
- In a large mixing bowl, combine the spinach, artichoke hearts, cream cheese, sour cream, mayonnaise, Parmesan cheese, garlic powder, salt, and pepper. Mix well.
- Transfer the mixture to an oven-safe baking dish.
- Bake for 20-25 minutes, or until the dip is hot and bubbly.
- Serve with tortilla chips, crackers, or veggies.

Nutrition Information (per serving):

Calories: 197

Fat: 18g

Carbohydrates: 5g

Protein: 6g

Fiber: 1g

Sodium: 338mg

Serving size: 1/4 cup

Note: This spinach and artichoke dip is a delicious and easy appetizer or snack. However, it is high in fat and sodium, so it's best enjoyed in moderation. To make it a little healthier, you can use low-fat or Greek yogurt instead of sour cream and mayonnaise, and serve it with veggies instead of chips or crackers. Enjoy!

7. Carrot and Ginger Dip

Ingredients:

- 2 medium carrots, peeled and chopped
- 1-inch piece of ginger, peeled and grated
- 1/2 cup plain Greek yogurt
- 1 tablespoon honey
- 1 tablespoon fresh lemon juice
- 1/4 teaspoon ground cumin
- Salt and pepper to taste

Nutritional Value:

Calories: 70

Fat: 1.5g

Carbohydrates: 11g

Fiber: 2g

Protein: 5g
Serving Size: Makes about 1 cup of dip, serving size is 2 tablespoons

Note: This dip is perfect for snacking or as a healthy topping for vegetables. It's low in calories and high in protein and fiber, making it a great option for anyone watching their weight or looking for a healthier snack. It's also a great way to get in your daily serving of vegetables!

8. Date and Nut Bars

Ingredients:

- 1 cup pitted dates
- 1 cup mixed nuts (almonds, cashews, pistachios, etc.)

- 1/4 cup honey
- 1/4 cup unsweetened coconut flakes
- 1 tsp vanilla extract
- 1/4 tsp sea salt

Directions:

- Preheat the oven to 350°F and line a baking dish with parchment paper.
- In a food processor, pulse the dates and mixed nuts until they form a sticky mixture.
- Add honey, coconut flakes, vanilla extract, and sea salt to the mixture and pulse until well combined.
- Transfer the mixture to the baking dish and press it down evenly with your hands or a spatula.
- Bake for 20-25 minutes or until lightly browned.

- Let cool for 10 minutes, then slice into bars.

Nutrition facts (per serving):

Calories: 195

Total fat: 9.5g

Saturated fat: 2.8g

Cholesterol: 0mg

Sodium: 67mg

Total carbohydrates: 27.5g

Dietary fiber: 3.5g

Sugars: 21.1g

Protein: 4.4g

Serving size: 1 bar

Note: These date and nut bars make a great healthy snack or breakfast option. They are high in fiber and protein, which helps to keep you full and satisfied. You can also customize the recipe by adding different nuts or dried fruits to the mixture. Store the bars in an airtight container in the fridge for up to a week.

9. Peanut Butter and Banana Bars

Ingredients:

- 2 ripe bananas, mashed
- 1/2 cup natural peanut butter
- 1/4 cup honey
- 2 cups rolled oats
- 1/2 cup chopped peanuts
- 1/4 tsp salt

Instructions:

- Preheat the oven to 350°F (175°C) and line an 8x8-inch baking dish with parchment paper.
- In a large mixing bowl, mix the mashed bananas, peanut butter, and honey until smooth.
- Add the rolled oats, chopped peanuts, and salt to the bowl, and stir until everything is well combined.
- Press the mixture evenly into the prepared baking dish and bake for 20-25 minutes or until the edges are golden brown.
- Let the bars cool in the dish for 10-15 minutes before slicing into 8 bars.
- Store the bars in an airtight container in the fridge for up to 1 week.

Nutritional Value:

Here's the approximate nutritional information for one serving (1 bar) of these Peanut Butter and Banana Bars:

Calories: 271

Total Fat: 13.3g

Saturated Fat: 2.3g

Cholesterol: 0mg

Sodium: 97mg

Total Carbohydrates: 33.3g

Dietary Fiber: 4.8g

Sugars: 14.2g

Protein: 8.5g

Serving Size:

This recipe makes 8 bars, and the serving size is 1 bar.

Note:

You can also customize this recipe by adding different mix-ins like chocolate chips or dried fruit. Additionally, you can substitute the peanut butter for other nut butters like almond or cashew butter if you have a preference or allergy.

10. Almond and Coconut Bars

Ingredients:

- 1 cup almond flour
- 1/2 cup unsweetened shredded coconut
- 1/4 cup melted coconut oil
- 1/4 cup honey
- 1 tsp vanilla extract

- 1/4 tsp sea salt

Instructions:

- Preheat oven to 350°F and line an 8x8 inch baking dish with parchment paper.
- In a large bowl, mix together almond flour and shredded coconut.
- In a separate bowl, whisk together melted coconut oil, honey, vanilla extract, and sea salt.
- Add the wet mixture to the dry mixture and stir until fully combined.
- Press the mixture firmly into the lined baking dish.
- Bake for 18-20 minutes, until the edges are golden brown.
- Let the bars cool completely before cutting into 12 equal pieces.

Nutritional Information (per serving):

Calories: 162

Fat: 13g

Carbohydrates: 10g

Fiber: 2g

Protein: 3g

Note: These bars can be stored in an airtight container in the fridge for up to a week. They make a great on-the-go snack or breakfast option. Feel free to add in other ingredients like chocolate chips or chopped nuts to customize to your liking.

Chapter 6

1. Berry Parfait

Ingredients:

- 1 cup plain Greek yogurt
- 1/2 cup mixed berries (strawberries, blueberries, raspberries)
- 1/4 cup granola
- 1 tablespoon honey (optional)

Directions:

- Wash and cut the berries into small pieces.

- In a small bowl, mix the Greek yogurt with honey (if using).

- In a glass, layer the yogurt, granola, and mixed berries.

- Repeat the layers until the glass is full.

- Serve and enjoy!

Nutritional Value per serving (1 parfait):

Calories: 272

Fat: 7g

Carbohydrates: 36g

Protein: 16g

Sugar: 19g

Fiber: 5g

Serving Size: 1 parfait

Note: This Berry Parfait is a healthy and delicious breakfast or snack option. It is high in protein, fiber, and antioxidants from the mixed berries. You can also swap the granola for chopped nuts for added crunch and healthy fats. Enjoy!

2. Banana Bread

Ingredients:

- 2-3 ripe bananas, mashed
- 1/3 cup melted butter
- 1 teaspoon baking soda
- Pinch of salt
- 3/4 cup sugar
- 1 large egg, beaten
- 1 teaspoon vanilla extract

- 1 1/2 cups all-purpose flour

Instructions:

- Preheat the oven to 350°F (175°C) and butter a 4x8-inch loaf pan.
- In a mixing bowl, combine the mashed bananas and melted butter.
- Add the baking soda and salt, then mix in the sugar, beaten egg, and vanilla extract.
- Add the flour and mix until just incorporated.
- Pour the batter into the prepared loaf pan and bake for 50-60 minutes, or until a toothpick inserted into the center of the bread comes out clean.
- Allow the bread to cool before slicing and serving.

Nutritional Value:

Serving Size: 1 slice (1/12 of loaf)

Calories: 170

Total Fat: 6g

Saturated Fat: 4g

Cholesterol: 29mg

Sodium: 206mg

Total Carbohydrates: 27g

Dietary Fiber: 1g

Sugars: 14g

Protein: 2g

Note:

This banana bread recipe is a classic, and the perfect way to use up overripe bananas. It's easy to make and perfect for breakfast, a snack, or dessert. Plus, it's relatively low in calories and fat compared to many other sweet treats. Just be sure to stick to the recommended serving size to keep your portions in check!

3. **Dark Chocolate Avocado Pudding**

Ingredients:

- 2 ripe avocados
- 1/2 cup unsweetened cocoa powder
- 1/4 cup honey or maple syrup
- 1/4 cup almond milk
- 1 tsp vanilla extract
- Pinch of salt
- Optional toppings: sliced bananas, strawberries, whipped cream, or chopped nuts

Directions:

- Cut the avocados in half, remove the pit and scoop out the flesh into a blender or food processor.
- Add the cocoa powder, honey or maple syrup, almond milk, vanilla extract, and salt.
- Blend until smooth and creamy.
- Serve in small cups or bowls and add your favorite toppings if desired.

Nutritional Information (per serving, without toppings):

Calories: 224

Total fat: 14g

Saturated fat: 3g

Cholesterol: 0mg

Sodium: 60mg

Total carbohydrates: 28g

Dietary fiber: 8g

Sugars: 16g

Protein: 4g

Serving size: Makes about 4 servings (1/2 cup each)

Note: This delicious and healthy dessert is a great way to satisfy your sweet tooth while also getting the health benefits of avocados. Avocados are a good source of healthy fats, fiber, vitamins, and minerals. This recipe is also gluten-free and dairy-free, making it a great option for those with food allergies or sensitivities. Enjoy!

4. Chia Seed Pudding

Ingredients:

- 1/2 cup chia seeds

- 2 cups almond milk

- 2-3 tablespoons honey or maple syrup

- 1 teaspoon vanilla extract

- Fresh fruit, nuts, or granola for topping

Directions:

- In a bowl, mix together chia seeds, almond milk, honey or maple syrup, and vanilla extract.

- Stir well and let sit for 5-10 minutes.

- Stir again and let sit for at least 30 minutes or overnight in the refrigerator.

- Serve in a bowl and add toppings of your choice.

Nutritional Value:

Calories: 276

Fat: 14g

Carbohydrates: 28g

Fiber: 17g

Protein: 9g

Serving Size:

This recipe makes 4 servings.

Note:

Chia seeds are a great source of fiber, protein, and healthy fats. They also have antioxidant properties and can help regulate blood sugar levels. This pudding makes for a healthy and satisfying breakfast or snack. You can customize the recipe by adding your favorite toppings or using different types of milk. Enjoy!

5. Coconut Macaroons

Ingredients:

- 14 oz sweetened shredded coconut
- 14 oz sweetened condensed milk
- 2 tsp vanilla extract
- 2 egg whites
- 1/4 tsp salt

Instructions:

- Preheat the oven to 350°F.
- In a large bowl, mix together the sweetened shredded coconut, sweetened condensed milk, and vanilla extract until well combined.
- In a separate bowl, beat the egg whites and salt until stiff peaks form.

- Fold the egg whites into the coconut mixture until fully incorporated.
- Using a cookie scoop or tablespoon, drop the coconut mixture onto a lined baking sheet.
- Bake for 20-25 minutes, or until golden brown.
- Let the macaroons cool on the baking sheet for 5 minutes before transferring to a wire rack to cool completely.

Nutritional Information (per serving - 1 macaroon):

Calories: 120
Fat: 6g
Saturated Fat: 5g
Cholesterol: 5mg
Sodium: 70mg

Carbohydrates: 15g

Fiber: 1g

Sugar: 13g

Protein: 2g

Serving Size: Makes approximately 28 macaroons

Note: These macaroons are gluten-free and can be made dairy-free by using a dairy-free sweetened condensed milk. They are a delicious and easy dessert or snack, perfect for those with a sweet tooth!

6. Oatmeal and Raisin Cookies

Ingredients:

- 1 cup all-purpose flour
- 1/2 teaspoon baking soda

- 1/2 teaspoon ground cinnamon
- 1/4 teaspoon salt
- 1/2 cup unsalted butter, softened
- 1/2 cup brown sugar
- 1/4 cup granulated sugar
- 1 large egg
- 1 teaspoon vanilla extract
- 1 1/2 cups old-fashioned oats
- 1/2 cup raisins

Instructions:

- Preheat oven to 350°F (180°C).
- In a medium bowl, whisk together the flour, baking soda, cinnamon, and salt.
- In a large mixing bowl, beat the butter, brown sugar, and granulated sugar together until light and fluffy.

- Add the egg and vanilla and mix until well combined.
- Gradually add the flour mixture to the butter mixture, mixing until just combined.
- Stir in the oats and raisins.
- Using a cookie scoop or spoon, drop dough onto a baking sheet lined with parchment paper.
- Bake for 10-12 minutes, or until the edges are lightly golden.
- Allow the cookies to cool on the baking sheet for 5 minutes before transferring them to a wire rack to cool completely.

Nutritional value:

Serving size: 1 cookie

Calories: 110

Fat: 5g

Carbohydrates: 15g

Protein: 2g

Fiber: 1g

Sugar: 7g

Note:

Oatmeal and raisin cookies can be stored in an airtight container at room temperature for up to 5 days. They also freeze well for up to 3 months. Enjoy these cookies as a snack or dessert, but be sure to enjoy them in moderation as they do contain sugar and fat.

7. Quinoa Banana Bread

Ingredients:

- 1 cup cooked quinoa

- 2 ripe bananas, mashed
- 2 eggs
- 1/3 cup honey
- 1/4 cup melted coconut oil
- 1 tsp vanilla extract
- 1 1/2 cups whole wheat flour
- 1 tsp baking powder
- 1/2 tsp baking soda
- 1/2 tsp salt
- 1/2 tsp ground cinnamon

Directions:

- Preheat oven to 350°F. Grease a 9x5 inch loaf pan with coconut oil.
- In a large bowl, whisk together cooked quinoa, mashed bananas, eggs, honey, coconut oil, and vanilla extract.

- In another bowl, mix together whole wheat flour, baking powder, baking soda, salt, and cinnamon.
- Add dry ingredients to wet ingredients and mix until just combined.
- Pour batter into prepared loaf pan and bake for 50-60 minutes or until a toothpick inserted into the center comes out clean.
- Allow bread to cool in the pan for 10 minutes before removing and transferring to a wire rack to cool completely.

Nutritional Information:

Servings: 10
Calories per serving: 214
Total fat: 8.6g
Total carbohydrates: 33.2g

Dietary fiber: 3.7g

Sugars: 15.9g

Protein: 5.2g

Note: This Quinoa Banana Bread is a healthy and delicious way to start your day. It's perfect for breakfast or as a snack. The addition of quinoa makes this bread high in protein and fiber, while the bananas add natural sweetness. Plus, it's easy to make and can be stored in the fridge or freezer for later enjoyment. Enjoy!

8. Spelt Flour Pumpkin Muffins

Ingredients:

- 2 cups spelt flour
- 1 teaspoon baking powder
- 1 teaspoon baking soda
- 1 teaspoon ground cinnamon
- 1/2 teaspoon ground nutmeg
- 1/2 teaspoon salt
- 1 cup canned pumpkin puree
- 1/2 cup honey
- 1/3 cup vegetable oil
- 2 eggs
- 1/4 cup milk
- 1 teaspoon vanilla extract

Instructions:

- Preheat the oven to 375°F (190°C) and line a muffin tin with paper liners.

- In a large bowl, whisk together the spelt flour, baking powder, baking soda, cinnamon, nutmeg, and salt.

- In a separate bowl, mix together the pumpkin puree, honey, vegetable oil, eggs, milk, and vanilla extract.

- Add the wet ingredients to the dry ingredients and stir until just combined.

- Divide the batter evenly among the muffin cups.

- Bake for 20-25 minutes or until a toothpick inserted in the center of a muffin comes out clean.

- Allow the muffins to cool in the tin for 5 minutes before transferring them to a wire rack to cool completely.

Nutritional Information (per serving - 1 muffin):

Calories: 182

Total Fat: 7g

Saturated Fat: 1g

Cholesterol: 35mg

Sodium: 226mg

Total Carbohydrates: 28g

Dietary Fiber: 3g

Sugars: 14g

Protein: 4g

Serving Size: 1 muffin

Note: Spelt flour is an ancient grain that is a good source of fiber and protein. It has a slightly nutty flavor and can be used as a substitute for regular wheat flour in many recipes. These spelt flour pumpkin muffins are a healthier alternative to traditional muffins, and they make a delicious breakfast or snack. Enjoy!

9. Dark Chocolate Avocado Brownies

Ingredients:

- 2 ripe avocados
- 1/2 cup maple syrup
- 1/2 cup unsweetened cocoa powder
- 3 eggs
- 1 tsp vanilla extract
- 1/2 tsp baking soda
- 1/4 tsp salt
- 1/2 cup dark chocolate chips

Instructions:

- Preheat the oven to 350°F (175°C).
- Peel and mash the avocados in a mixing bowl.
- Add maple syrup, cocoa powder, eggs, vanilla extract, baking soda, and salt. Mix well.
- Stir in the dark chocolate chips.
- Pour the mixture into a greased 8x8 inch baking dish.
- Bake for 25-30 minutes, or until a toothpick comes out clean when inserted in the center.
- Let cool for at least 10 minutes before serving.

Nutritional Value (per serving):

Calories: 226

Fat: 14.2g

Carbohydrates: 26.4g

Fiber: 5.5g

Protein: 5g

Serving Size:

This recipe makes 9 brownies. One serving is one brownie.

Note:

Avocado is a great source of healthy fats and fiber, making it a nutritious ingredient for brownies. Dark chocolate is also rich in antioxidants and may have heart-healthy benefits. These brownies are a healthier alternative to traditional brownies, but should still be consumed in moderation.

10. Beetroot Chocolate Cake

Ingredients:

- 2 medium beetroots, cooked and pureed
- 1 cup all-purpose flour
- 1/2 cup unsweetened cocoa powder
- 1 tsp baking powder
- 1 tsp baking soda
- 1/2 tsp salt
- 3/4 cup sugar
- 1/3 cup vegetable oil
- 2 eggs
- 1 tsp vanilla extract
- 1/2 cup milk
- Optional: chocolate chips or nuts for topping

Nutritional value (per serving):

Calories: 215

Protein: 4g

Fat: 10g

Carbohydrates: 30g

Fiber: 3g

Sugar: 17g

Sodium: 232mg

Serving size: 12 slices

Note: This cake is a healthier alternative to traditional chocolate cake as it contains pureed beetroots which are a good source of fiber, folate, and potassium. The cake is also lower in sugar and fat compared to other chocolate cakes. Enjoy this delicious and nutritious cake as a treat or a dessert with your family and friends!

Chapter 7

Sample meal plans for a week
Monday:

Breakfast: Oatmeal with berries and almond milk

Snack: Hard boiled egg and apple slices

Lunch: Grilled chicken salad with avocado and mixed greens

Snack: Carrots and hummus

Dinner: Salmon with roasted sweet potato and broccoli

Tuesday:

Breakfast: Greek yogurt with granola and mixed berries
Snack: Almonds and pear slices
Lunch: Quinoa salad with grilled vegetables and feta cheese
Snack: Edamame
Dinner: Turkey meatballs with spaghetti squash and marinara sauce

Wednesday:

Breakfast: Whole wheat toast with almond butter and banana slices

Snack: String cheese and orange slices

Lunch: Lentil soup with mixed greens salad

Snack: Roasted chickpeas

Dinner: Grilled shrimp with brown rice and asparagus

Thursday:

Breakfast: Scrambled eggs with spinach and whole wheat toast

Snack: Trail mix

Lunch: Tuna salad with mixed greens and whole wheat crackers

Snack: Green smoothie

Dinner: Grilled steak with roasted Brussels sprouts and sweet potato fries

Friday:

Breakfast: Smoothie bowl with Greek yogurt, mixed berries, and granola

Snack: Cottage cheese and peach slices

Lunch: Roasted vegetable wrap with avocado and hummus

Snack: Dark chocolate and almonds

Dinner: Grilled chicken with quinoa and roasted vegetables

Saturday:

Breakfast: Whole wheat pancakes with mixed berries and honey

Snack: Apple slices with almond butter

Lunch: Grilled salmon with mixed greens and quinoa salad

Snack: Greek yogurt with honey and walnuts

Dinner: Roasted vegetable lasagna with whole wheat noodles

Sunday:

Breakfast: Egg and vegetable frittata with whole wheat toast

Snack: Trail mix

Lunch: Grilled chicken and vegetable kebabs with quinoa salad

Snack: Apple slices with peanut butter

Dinner: Turkey chili with mixed greens salad and whole wheat crackers.

Tips for meal planning and preparation

1. Plan your meals in advance.
2. Choose a variety of fruits and vegetables.
3. Incorporate whole grains into your diet.
4. Use lean protein sources such as chicken, fish, and beans.
5. Avoid processed foods.
6. Limit your intake of sugar and refined carbohydrates.
7. Drink plenty of water.
8. Avoid alcohol and caffeine.
9. Choose healthy fats such as avocado and nuts.

10. Use herbs and spices to add flavor to your meals.

11. Don't skip breakfast.

12. Include healthy snacks in your meal plan.

13. Meal prep on the weekends to save time during the week.

14. Use a slow cooker to prepare meals ahead of time.

15. Keep healthy snacks on hand for when you're on the go.

16. Cook in bulk and freeze leftovers for future meals.

17. Shop for groceries with a list to avoid impulse buying.

18. Choose organic and non-GMO foods when possible.

19. Avoid artificial sweeteners and colors.

20. Use a food scale to measure portion sizes.

21.Read food labels to ensure you're getting the nutrients you need.

22. Choose low-fat dairy products.

23. Incorporate probiotics into your diet.

24. Choose plant-based protein sources such as tofu and tempeh.

25. Avoid fried foods and instead bake, broil, or grill your meals.

26. Use a meal delivery service to save time and ensure healthy options.

27. Incorporate leafy greens into your diet.

28. Choose healthy carbohydrates such as quinoa and sweet potatoes.

29. Limit your intake of red meat.

30. Avoid processed meats such as bacon and sausage.

31. Incorporate healthy oils such as olive and coconut oil.

32. Don't rely on takeout or restaurant meals for your nutrition.

33. Plan meals that are high in antioxidants.

34. Choose foods high in folic acid.

35. Incorporate iron-rich foods such as spinach and lentils.

36. Avoid high mercury fish such as shark and swordfish.

37. Choose seafood with low mercury levels such as salmon and sardines.

38. Incorporate nuts and seeds into your diet.

39. Use a food journal to track what you eat.

40. Don't skip meals or restrict calories.

41. Choose high fiber foods such as beans and whole grains.

42. Incorporate fermented foods such as kefir and sauerkraut.

43. Choose colorful fruits and vegetables for a variety of nutrients.

44. Avoid foods with added hormones or antibiotics.

45. Choose foods high in vitamin D.

46. Incorporate whole food sources of calcium.

47. Choose lean cuts of meat such as chicken breast and turkey.

48. Use healthy cooking methods such as steaming and baking.

49. Incorporate healthy carbs such as brown rice and quinoa.

50. Limit your intake of processed snacks such as chips and crackers.

51. Choose healthy sweeteners such as honey and maple syrup.

52. Avoid high-calorie drinks such as soda and juice.

53. Choose foods high in vitamin E.

54. Incorporate healthy fats such as chia seeds and flaxseeds.

55. Limit your intake of saturated fats.

56. Choose whole food sources of iron.

57. Incorporate foods high in vitamin C.

58. Use a pressure cooker to save time when meal prepping.

59. Choose foods high in zinc.

60. Incorporate healthy carbs such as oats and barley.

61. Limit your intake of high-sugar foods such as candy and pastries.

62. Choose foods high in vitamin A.

63. Incorporate healthy fats such as salmon and avocado.

64. Use portion control to ensure you're not overeating.

65. Choose foods high in selenium.

66. Incorporate healthy

Conclusion

Final thoughts on the fertility diet

The fertility diet is a healthy eating pattern that emphasizes whole foods, fruits, vegetables, whole grains, and healthy fats while minimizing intake of processed and refined foods, red meat, and sugary drinks. It has been associated with improved fertility outcomes, including higher chances of conception, reduced risk of ovulatory infertility, and better pregnancy outcomes.

The fertility diet's focus on healthy, nutrient-dense foods can improve overall health and reduce the risk of chronic diseases such as obesity, diabetes, and heart disease. However, it is not a magical solution and should not be viewed as a substitute for medical advice or fertility treatments.

It is essential to consult a healthcare professional and undergo regular check-ups to address any underlying health issues that may affect fertility. Additionally, lifestyle factors such as physical activity, stress management, and adequate sleep should also be considered alongside the fertility diet.

Overall, following a healthy eating pattern such as the fertility diet, along with a healthy lifestyle, can improve overall health and increase the chances of conception for couples trying to conceive.

www.ingramcontent.com/pod-product-compliance
Lightning Source LLC
Chambersburg PA
CBHW071219260726
48653CB00042B/1313